HAIR CARE

TREATMENT FOR HAIR LOSS

ROSIE PHILIP

TABLE OF CONTENTS

GENTLE WASHING

Gentle washing is a crucial aspect of hair care, particularly for those dealing with hair loss or looking to maintain overall hair health. In this detailed exploration, we will delve into the significance of gentle washing, the best practices, and the impact it has on the health and appearance of your hair.

Hair is a delicate structure composed of protein strands, primarily keratin. The scalp, where hair follicles reside, produces natural oils (sebum) that contribute to hair health. Gentle washing plays a pivotal role in preserving these natural oils while effectively cleansing the hair and scalp.

The importance of gentle washing

 It's essential to recognize the potential harm caused by harsh cleansing practices. Many commercial shampoos contain sulfates, aggressive detergents that strip the hair and scalp of their natural oils. While these detergents create a rich lather and give the feeling of a thorough cleanse, they can also lead to dryness, frizz, and weakened hair strands.

When it comes to hair loss, the significance of gentle washing becomes even more apparent. Hair follicles are sensitive structures, and excessive washing with harsh products can cause inflammation and damage, leading to increased hair shedding. Moreover, for individuals experiencing conditions like androgenetic alopecia or telogen effluvium, preserving the health of existing hair becomes paramount.

Choosing a sulfate-free shampoo is a foundational step towards gentle washing. Sulfate-free formulations are milder on the hair and scalp, ensuring effective cleaning without the detrimental effects associated with sulfates. These shampoos often contain alternative cleansers like cocamidopropyl betaine, derived from coconut oil, providing a gentler cleansing experience.

In addition to selecting the right shampoo, the technique used during washing is equally crucial. Massaging the scalp with fingertips in gentle, circular motions promotes blood circulation, which is beneficial for hair follicle health. It also helps distribute natural oils evenly, preventing excessive dryness at the ends and maintaining a healthy scalp environment.

The frequency of washing is another aspect that varies among individuals. While some may benefit from daily washing, others may find it sufficient to wash their hair a few times a week. This depends on factors such as hair type, lifestyle, and individual preferences. Overwashing can lead to a loss of essential oils, while infrequent washing may result in a buildup of oils and styling products, potentially affecting the scalp's health.

For those with oily scalps, choosing a balancing shampoo and washing more frequently may be beneficial. On the other hand, individuals with dry or curly hair might benefit from less frequent washing and the use of hydrating products to maintain moisture.

It's important to note that the water temperature used during washing also contributes to the overall health of the hair. Hot water can strip the hair of natural oils, leaving it dry and more prone to breakage. Lukewarm or cool water is gentler on the hair and helps in retaining moisture.

Incorporating a pre-shampoo routine can enhance the benefits of gentle washing. Applying a natural oil, such as coconut or jojoba oil, to the hair before washing acts as a protective barrier, minimizing the impact of cleansing agents and providing additional nourishment. This pre-shampoo treatment can be especially beneficial for individuals with dry or damaged hair.

While gentle washing is crucial, the choice of conditioner is equally important in a haircare routine. Using a conditioner designed for your hair type and concerns helps in maintaining moisture, preventing tangles, and enhancing the overall manageability of the hair. Applying conditioner primarily to the ends of the hair and avoiding the scalp area can prevent excess buildup.

Gentle washing is a cornerstone of effective hair care, particularly for those dealing with hair loss or aiming to maintain healthy and vibrant hair. Choosing sulfate-free shampoos, employing proper washing techniques, adjusting washing frequency based on individual needs, and incorporating pre-shampoo treatments are all integral aspects of a gentle washing routine. By adopting these practices, individuals can nurture their hair, minimize damage, and contribute to an environment conducive to optimal hair health.

SCALP MASSAGE

Scalp massage, often considered a luxurious and relaxing practice, goes beyond its soothing effects; it can significantly contribute to the overall health of the hair and scalp. In this comprehensive exploration, we will delve into the intricacies of scalp massage, its numerous benefits, the techniques involved, and how incorporating this ritual into your routine can promote not only relaxation but also optimal hair growth and health.

The Significance of Scalp Health

The scalp is the foundation of hair health. It houses hair follicles, sebaceous glands, and blood vessels, all crucial components in the hair growth process. A healthy scalp is essential for ensuring strong, vibrant hair. However, various factors such as stress, environmental pollutants, and improper care practices can negatively impact scalp health, leading to issues like dryness, flakiness, and even hair loss.

Understanding Scalp Massage
Scalp massage is a therapeutic technique involving the manipulation of the scalp using various movements, pressure levels, and sometimes, specific oils. This practice has been a part of traditional cultures for centuries, with roots in Ayurveda, Chinese medicine, and other holistic approaches to well-being.

Benefits of Scalp Massage

Increased Blood Circulation: One of the primary benefits of scalp massage is the promotion of blood circulation. The gentle pressure applied during a massage stimulates blood flow to the scalp, bringing with it oxygen and essential nutrients. Improved circulation nourishes hair follicles, supporting their health and function.

Relaxation and Stress Reduction: Scalp massage induces relaxation by easing tension in the muscles and reducing stress levels. Stress is a known contributor to hair loss, and incorporating regular scalp massages into your routine can be an effective way to manage stress and potentially mitigate its impact on your hair.

Enhanced Nutrient Delivery: By improving blood circulation, scalp massage facilitates the efficient delivery of nutrients to the hair follicles. This is crucial for the production of healthy hair strands. Nutrient-rich blood encourages the follicles to function optimally, promoting robust and lustrous hair growth.

Oil Distribution: The sebaceous glands in the scalp produce natural oils (sebum) that help moisturize and protect the hair. Scalp massage assists in distributing these oils along the hair shaft, preventing dryness at the roots and promoting a healthy shine.

Exfoliation: The massaging action helps in the removal of dead skin cells, excess oils, and product buildup from the scalp. This gentle exfoliation promotes a clean and healthy scalp environment, reducing the risk of issues like dandruff and itching.

Techniques for Effective Scalp Massage

Circular Motion: Using your fingertips, apply gentle circular motions across the scalp. Begin at the forehead and work your way backward. This technique stimulates blood flow and promotes relaxation.

Kneading: Lift small sections of hair and gently knead the scalp using your fingertips. This helps release tension in specific areas and enhances the overall massage experience.

Tapping or Drumming: Lightly tap your fingertips on the scalp, moving across the entire area. This technique can invigorate the scalp and improve blood circulation.

Pressure Points: Incorporate pressure point massage by applying gentle pressure to specific points on the scalp. This can enhance the therapeutic effects of the massage and alleviate tension.

Oil Massage: Using natural oils like coconut, jojoba, or almond oil during a scalp massage can add an extra layer of nourishment. Apply the oil to your fingertips and distribute it evenly across the scalp while massaging.

Integrating Scalp Massage into Your Routine
Incorporating scalp massage into your routine doesn't have to be time-consuming. Even a few minutes a few times a week can yield noticeable benefits. You can perform scalp massage during your regular shower, before bedtime, or as part of a pampering self-care session.

Pre-Shampoo Ritual: Consider incorporating scalp massage as a pre-shampoo ritual. Apply a small amount of oil to your scalp, massage for a few minutes, and then proceed with your regular hair washing routine. This not only enhances the massage experience but also adds a nourishing element to your hair care routine.

Use Massage Tools: Scalp massage can be amplified with the use of various tools, such as scalp massage brushes or handheld massagers. These tools can provide additional stimulation and make the massage process more enjoyable.

Mindful Relaxation: Take advantage of scalp massage as a time for mindfulness and relaxation. Focus on the sensations, and allow yourself to unwind. Combining relaxation techniques with scalp massage can maximize its stress-relieving benefits.

A scalp massage is not merely a luxurious indulgence but a practical and effective way to promote scalp health and support optimal hair growth. Its benefits extend beyond relaxation, encompassing improved blood circulation, stress reduction, enhanced nutrient delivery, oil distribution, and gentle exfoliation. By understanding the significance of scalp health and incorporating regular massages into your routine, you can contribute to the overall well-being of your hair and indulge in a self-care practice that nurtures both your scalp and your mind.

NUTRIENT-DENSE DIET

A nutrient-rich diet is a cornerstone of promoting overall health, and its impact extends to the health and vitality of our hair. In this in-depth exploration, we will delve into the significance of a nutrient-rich diet for maintaining optimal hair health, the key nutrients involved, and practical dietary strategies to support hair growth and prevent issues such as hair loss and brittleness.

The Importance of Nutrition for Hair Health

The health of our hair is intricately linked to the nutrients we consume. Hair is composed of a protein called keratin, and various vitamins, minerals, and other compounds play essential roles in supporting its growth, strength, and overall condition. When our bodies lack these crucial nutrients, it can manifest in various hair-related issues, including thinning, dullness, and even hair loss.

Key Nutrients for Healthy Hair

Protein: Protein is the building block of hair, and ensuring an adequate intake is vital for maintaining strong and healthy strands. Foods rich in protein, such as lean meats, fish, eggs, dairy products, legumes, and nuts, should be integral components of a nutrient-rich diet.

Iron: Iron is essential for proper circulation, and inadequate levels can lead to hair loss. Incorporate iron-rich foods like red meat, poultry, fish, lentils, and leafy greens to support both overall health and hair growth.

Vitamins A and E: These vitamins are antioxidants that contribute to a healthy scalp. Foods like sweet potatoes, carrots, spinach, almonds, and sunflower seeds are excellent sources of these vitamins.

Vitamin D: Vitamin D is crucial for hair follicle cycling. Exposure to sunlight, fortified foods, fatty fish, and egg yolks are ways to ensure sufficient vitamin D intake.

B Vitamins (Biotin, B12, Niacin): B vitamins play a key role in promoting hair growth and preventing hair loss. Foods like eggs, nuts, seeds, dairy products, and leafy greens provide a rich supply of these essential nutrients.

Omega-3 Fatty Acids: Found in fatty fish, flaxseeds, chia seeds, and walnuts, omega-3 fatty acids contribute to scalp health, prevent dryness, and add shine to the hair.

Zinc: Zinc deficiency can lead to hair shedding. Foods such as oysters, beef, pumpkin seeds, and lentils are good sources of zinc.

Copper: Copper helps in the formation of melanin, the pigment responsible for hair color. Nuts, seeds, whole grains, and seafood are rich in copper.

Dietary Strategies for Healthy Hair

Balanced Diet: Aim for a well-rounded, balanced diet that includes a variety of fruits, vegetables, whole grains, lean proteins, and healthy fats. This ensures a diverse range of nutrients necessary for overall health and hair vitality.

Protein-Rich Foods: Incorporate adequate protein into your diet. Include sources such as poultry, fish, eggs, legumes, and plant-based protein alternatives to meet your daily protein requirements.

Iron Absorption: Enhance iron absorption by combining iron-rich foods with sources of vitamin C. For example, pair spinach (iron-rich) with strawberries (vitamin C) in a salad.

Omega-3 Fatty Acids: Consume fatty fish like salmon, mackerel, or sardines at least twice a week to ensure an ample supply of omega-3 fatty acids. Vegetarian sources include flaxseeds, chia seeds, and walnuts.

Hydration: Stay adequately hydrated, as water is essential for overall bodily functions, including hair health. Dehydration can lead to dry and brittle hair.

Limit Processed Foods: Reduce the intake of processed and sugary foods, as they can contribute to inflammation and negatively impact overall health, including the health of hair follicles.

Supplements: In some cases, supplements may be necessary to fill nutritional gaps. Consult with a healthcare professional before incorporating any supplements into your routine.

Avoid Crash Diets: Extreme diets or rapid weight loss can deprive the body of essential nutrients, leading to hair loss. Focus on gradual, sustainable changes for long-term health benefits.

Practical Tips for Incorporating Nutrient-Rich Foods

Colorful Plate: Aim for a colorful plate with a variety of fruits and vegetables. The different colors often indicate a diverse range of vitamins and minerals.

Meal Planning: Plan meals in advance to ensure a balanced intake of nutrients throughout the day. Include a mix of protein, carbohydrates, and healthy fats.

Snack Smart: Choose nutrient-dense snacks such as Greek yogurt with berries, a handful of nuts, or vegetable sticks with hummus to boost your daily nutrient intake.

Herbs and Spices: Use herbs and spices to add flavor to your dishes. Many herbs and spices also offer additional health benefits.

Rotate Foods: Rotate your food choices to ensure a broad spectrum of nutrients. Eating the same foods every day may lead to nutrient imbalances.

A nutrient-rich diet is not only crucial for overall health but also plays a pivotal role in promoting vibrant, healthy hair. By prioritizing foods rich in protein, vitamins, minerals, and essential fatty acids, individuals can support the strength, growth, and appearance of their hair. The holistic approach to hair health through nutrition not only addresses specific concerns but also contributes to overall well-being. It's important to recognize that consistency in a nutrient-rich diet, coupled with a healthy lifestyle, forms the foundation for maintaining beautiful and resilient hair throughout life.

AVOID HEAT STYLING

Avoiding heat styling is a fundamental aspect of maintaining healthy hair. In this detailed exploration, we will delve into the reasons why heat styling can be detrimental, the potential damage it can cause, and practical alternatives and tips for achieving stylish looks without subjecting your hair to excessive heat.

Understanding Heat Damage
Heat styling tools such as flat irons, curling irons, and blow dryers can significantly impact the health of your hair. The high temperatures generated by these tools can strip the hair of its natural moisture, leading to dryness, breakage, and overall damage. The three main types of heat damage are:

Structural Damage: Excessive heat can break down the protein structure of the hair, leading to weakened and brittle strands.

Moisture Loss: High temperatures can evaporate the natural moisture present in the hair, resulting in dryness and a lack of elasticity.

Cuticle Damage: The outer layer of the hair, the cuticle, can suffer damage from heat styling, leading to raised cuticles, frizz, and a compromised protective barrier.

The Impact of Heat Styling on Hair Health

Dryness and Brittle Hair: Frequent use of heat styling tools can deplete the hair's natural moisture, leaving it dry and prone to breakage. This dryness can make the hair appear dull and lifeless.

Split Ends: Heat styling can contribute to split ends, where the hair shaft splits into two or more parts. This not only affects the appearance of the hair but also compromises its overall health.

Loss of Shine: The cuticle damage caused by heat styling can lead to a loss of the hair's natural shine. Dull and lackluster hair is a common consequence of regular heat exposure.

Reduced Elasticity: The loss of moisture and structural damage can reduce the hair's elasticity, making it more susceptible to breakage and less capable of withstanding tension.

Color Fading: For individuals with color-treated hair, heat styling can accelerate color fading, leading to the need for more frequent touch-ups.

Alternatives to Heat Styling

Air Drying: Allow your hair to air dry naturally instead of using a blow dryer. This gentler method minimizes exposure to heat and helps retain the hair's natural moisture.

Heatless Curling Techniques: Achieve curls without heat by using techniques such as braiding, twisting, or using heatless curlers. These methods are not only heat-free but can also create beautiful, natural-looking curls.

Twist Outs and Braid Outs: Create defined waves or curls by twisting or braiding damp hair before bedtime. In the morning, unravel the twists or braids for heat-free styling.

Roller Sets: Use roller sets for volume and curls without the need for heat. Velcro or foam rollers can be applied to damp hair, and once dry, they provide a bouncy and heat-free styling option.

Protective Styles: Opt for protective styles like braids, twists, or buns, which not only reduce the need for daily styling but also shield the hair from external elements.

Wet Sets: Utilize wet sets, such as flexi rods or perm rods, to achieve curls without heat. These sets can be done on damp hair and left to air dry.

Tips for Minimizing Heat Damage

Use Heat Protectant: When heat styling is unavoidable, use a quality heat protectant spray or serum. This creates a protective barrier between the hair and the heat, minimizing damage.

Adjust Heat Settings: If using heat styling tools, adjust the temperature settings based on your hair type. Lower heat settings are suitable for finer or more delicate hair, reducing the risk of damage.

Limit Frequency: Minimize the frequency of heat styling. Allowing your hair to rest from heat exposure can significantly contribute to its overall health.

Invest in Quality Tools: High-quality heat styling tools with advanced technology and ceramic or tourmaline plates can distribute heat more evenly, reducing the risk of hot spots and excessive damage.

Prevent Overlapping: When using a flat iron or curling iron, avoid overlapping sections of hair, as this can lead to uneven heat distribution and increased damage.

Regular Trims: Schedule regular trims to remove split ends and prevent further damage. Trimming is essential for maintaining the overall health and appearance of the hair.

Deep Conditioning: Incorporate regular deep conditioning treatments into your hair care routine to replenish moisture and strengthen the hair shaft.

The Psychological Impact of Heat-Free Styling
Beyond the physical benefits of avoiding heat styling, there are psychological advantages to embracing one's natural hair texture. The pressure to conform to societal

beauty standards often promotes a certain image of sleek, straight, or perfectly styled hair. However, embracing your natural hair can foster self-acceptance and confidence.

Avoiding heat styling is a proactive approach to maintaining healthy, vibrant hair. The potential damage caused by excessive heat exposure is well-documented, and alternatives and tips for heat-free styling offer practical solutions for achieving stylish looks without compromising the health of your hair. By embracing heat-free styling techniques, adjusting styling habits, and prioritizing the overall health of your hair, you can enjoy beautiful, resilient locks that reflect your natural beauty.

DEEP CONDITIONING

Deep conditioning is a vital component of a comprehensive haircare routine, offering numerous benefits for maintaining healthy, vibrant hair. In this extensive exploration, we will delve into the significance of deep conditioning, the science behind it, the types of deep conditioners available, and practical tips for incorporating this nourishing treatment into your regular hair care regimen.

Understanding Deep Conditioning
Deep conditioning involves the use of specialized hair care products designed to penetrate the hair shaft and provide intense moisturization and nourishment. Unlike regular conditioners, which primarily focus on the surface of the hair, deep conditioners work at a deeper level, addressing issues such as dryness, damage, and overall hair health.

The Science of Deep Conditioning
Hair strands consist of an outer protective layer called the cuticle, beneath which is the cortex containing proteins, such as keratin. The cuticle, when healthy, lies flat, creating a smooth surface that reflects light and gives the hair its shine. However, various factors, including heat styling, chemical treatments, and environmental stressors, can lead to cuticle damage, resulting in dry and dull hair.

Deep conditioning products typically contain a blend of moisturizing ingredients, proteins, and sometimes oils that work synergistically to address specific hair concerns. These formulations are designed to:

Moisturize: Deep conditioners infuse the hair with moisture, helping to combat dryness and improve overall hydration. This is particularly beneficial for individuals with naturally dry or curly hair types.

Strengthen: Protein-rich deep conditioners contribute to the structural integrity of the hair, reinforcing the protein bonds within the cortex. This can enhance the strength and resilience of the hair strands.

Repair: Ingredients such as amino acids and ceramides in deep conditioners can repair damaged areas of the hair, including split ends and areas where the cuticle may be compromised.

Smooth and Detangle: Deep conditioning helps in smoothing the hair cuticle, reducing friction between strands, and facilitating easier detangling. This is especially valuable for individuals with coarse or textured hair.

Types of Deep Conditioners

Moisturizing Deep Conditioners: Formulated with ingredients like glycerin, aloe vera, and hyaluronic acid, these conditioners focus on providing intense hydration to combat dryness and improve overall moisture retention.

Protein-Based Deep Conditioners: Enriched with proteins such as keratin, collagen, or amino acids, these conditioners are designed to strengthen and repair damaged hair, particularly beneficial for those with chemically treated or heat-damaged hair.

Hybrid Deep Conditioners: Many products on the market combine both moisturizing and protein elements to offer a comprehensive treatment for a wide range of hair types and concerns.

Oil-Based Deep Conditioners: These conditioners often contain nourishing oils like coconut, argan, or jojoba oil to provide deep hydration and add a layer of protection to the hair.

Benefits of Deep Conditioning

Hydration: Deep conditioning infuses the hair with moisture, preventing dryness and improving overall hydration. Well-moisturized hair is more manageable, less prone to breakage, and exhibits a healthy shine.

Improved Elasticity: The proteins in deep conditioners contribute to the elasticity of the hair, making it more flexible and less prone to breakage. This is crucial for maintaining strong and resilient strands.

Enhanced Shine and Smoothness: Deep conditioning smoothens the hair cuticle, reducing friction between strands. This results in a smoother texture, enhanced shine, and improved overall manageability.

Prevention of Breakage: Regular deep conditioning helps prevent breakage by fortifying the hair strands, reducing brittleness, and addressing areas of damage. This is especially beneficial for individuals with chemically treated or heat-styled hair.

Color Protection: For those with color-treated hair, deep conditioning can help maintain vibrancy and prevent color fading. The added moisture and nourishment contribute to the longevity of the color.

How to Deep Condition Effectively

Pre-Shampoo vs. Post-Shampoo: Deep conditioning can be done either before or after shampooing. Pre-shampoo treatments are applied to dry hair before washing, while post-shampoo treatments are applied to clean, damp hair.

Application Techniques: Apply the deep conditioner evenly, focusing on mid-lengths and ends where the hair is usually drier and more prone to damage. Use a wide-tooth comb to ensure even distribution.

Processing Time: Follow the recommended processing time specified on the product label. Most deep conditioners require anywhere from 5 to 30 minutes, depending on the formulation and the level of treatment needed.

Heat Application: Applying heat can enhance the effectiveness of deep conditioning. Use a shower cap or warm towel to create a controlled environment that allows the product to penetrate the hair more deeply.

Frequency: The frequency of deep conditioning depends on factors such as hair type, condition, and the specific needs of your hair. While some individuals may benefit from weekly deep conditioning, others may find monthly treatments sufficient.

DIY Deep Conditioning: Homemade deep conditioning treatments using natural ingredients like avocado, honey, yogurt, or coconut oil can be effective. These DIY options can be tailored to address specific hair concerns.

Deep Conditioning and Hair Types

Curly and Coily Hair: Individuals with curly or coily hair often have drier hair due to the natural oils taking longer to travel down the hair shaft. Deep conditioning is crucial for maintaining moisture, defining curls, and preventing breakage.

Straight and Wavy Hair: While straight and wavy hair types may not require as much moisture as curly hair, they can still benefit from deep conditioning to address issues like damage from heat styling or chemical treatments.

Chemically Treated Hair: Hair that has undergone chemical treatments such as coloring, perming, or relaxing is more prone to damage. Deep conditioning is essential for restoring moisture and maintaining the health of chemically treated strands.

Deep conditioning is a key element in maintaining healthy, resilient hair. Whether your hair is naturally dry, curly, straight, or chemically treated, incorporating deep conditioning into your regular hair care routine can provide a range of benefits, from improved hydration and elasticity to enhanced shine and color protection. Understanding the specific needs of your hair, choosing the right type of deep conditioner, and following effective application techniques are essential steps toward achieving optimal results. By making deep conditioning a consistent part of your hair care regimen, you can contribute to the overall health and beauty of your hair, ensuring it remains vibrant and strong.

AVOID TIGHT HAIRSTYLES

Avoiding tight hairstyles is a fundamental aspect of maintaining healthy hair. In this extensive exploration, we will delve into the reasons why tight hairstyles can be detrimental, the potential damage they can cause, and practical alternatives and tips for achieving stylish looks without subjecting your hair to unnecessary tension and stress.

Understanding the Impact of Tight Hairstyles
Hairstyles that exert excessive tension on the hair follicles and strands can lead to various issues, both short-term and long-term. The three primary areas of concern related to tight hairstyles are:

Traction Alopecia: This is a type of hair loss caused by constant pulling or tension on the hair. Tight hairstyles, such as tight ponytails, braids, or buns, can contribute to traction alopecia by putting undue stress on the hair follicles, leading to inflammation and eventual hair loss.

Breakage and Split Ends: Tightly pulled hairstyles can cause mechanical damage to the hair shaft, resulting in breakage and split ends. The excessive tension weakens the hair structure, making it more prone to breakage.

Scalp Issues: Tight hairstyles can contribute to scalp issues such as irritation, redness, and even conditions like folliculitis. The constant pulling can damage the hair follicles and affect the overall health of the scalp.

Types of Tight Hairstyles to Avoid

High Ponytails: Pulling the hair tightly into a high ponytail can lead to stress on the hairline and increased tension on the scalp.

Tight Braids and Cornrows: While braids and cornrows can be stylish, overly tight ones can lead to traction alopecia and damage to the hair shaft.

Buns and Topknots: Styles that involve twisting and securing the hair tightly into a bun or topknot can cause stress on the hair follicles.

Tight Headbands and Hair Accessories: Accessories that grip the hair tightly can contribute to hair loss, especially around the edges and temples.

The Impact of Tight Hairstyles on Different Hair Types

Curly and Coily Hair: Individuals with curly or coily hair may experience more visible damage from tight hairstyles, as their hair texture is naturally more prone to breakage.

Fine and Thin Hair: Fine and thin hair is generally more delicate and susceptible to breakage. Tight hairstyles can exacerbate this vulnerability, leading to increased hair loss.

Chemically Treated Hair: Hair that has undergone chemical treatments such as coloring, relaxing, or perming is already compromised. Tight hairstyles can further weaken chemically treated strands.

Alternatives to Tight Hairstyles

Loose Ponytails and Braids: Opt for loose ponytails or braids instead of tightly pulled styles. This reduces tension on the hair follicles while still providing a stylish look.

Messy Buns and Low Knots: Embrace the beauty of loose, messy buns or low knots. These styles offer a more relaxed and comfortable alternative to tight updos.

Twists and Twirls: Create twists or twirls that are not pulled tightly. This allows for a textured and stylish appearance without compromising hair health.

Half-Up Styles: Half-up hairstyles can be a great compromise, offering the convenience of having some hair pulled back without the excessive tension of a tightly secured style.

Hair Clips and Accessories: Use hair clips, barrettes, or other accessories to secure hair without pulling it tightly.

This allows for versatility in styling without compromising hair health.

Protective Styles: Consider protective styles that don't rely on excessive tension, such as loose braids, twists, or protective updos that distribute the weight evenly.

Tips for Protecting Your Hair

Choose the Right Hair Accessories: Opt for accessories that are gentle on the hair, such as fabric-covered elastic bands, soft scrunchies, or hairpins with smooth edges.

Avoid Styles That Cause Pain: If a hairstyle feels too tight or causes discomfort, it's best to loosen it or choose a different style altogether. Pain is often an indicator of excessive tension.

Rotate Hairstyles: Avoid consistently wearing the same tight hairstyle every day. Rotating hairstyles allows for even distribution of tension and minimizes the risk of constant stress on specific areas.

Protective Styling at Night: If you prefer to sleep with your hair secured, choose a loose braid or a satin/silk scarf or bonnet to protect your hair while minimizing tension.

Regular Scalp Massages: Incorporate regular scalp massages into your routine to stimulate blood circulation and promote a healthy scalp environment, especially if you often wear tight hairstyles.

Hydrate and Nourish: Keep your hair well-hydrated and nourished with regular deep conditioning treatments. Moisturized hair is more flexible and less prone to breakage.

The Psychological Impact of Hairstyles
Beyond the physical benefits of avoiding tight hairstyles, there are psychological advantages to embracing more relaxed styles. The societal pressure to conform to certain beauty standards often influences hairstyle choices. However, embracing a variety of styles that prioritize comfort and health over stringent aesthetics can positively impact one's self-perception and confidence.

Avoiding tight hairstyles is a proactive approach to maintaining healthy, vibrant hair. The potential damage caused by excessive tension and stress on the hair follicles and strands is well-documented, and alternatives and tips for gentle styling offer practical solutions for achieving stylish looks without compromising the health of your hair. By embracing loose and comfortable hairstyles, choosing the right accessories, and prioritizing the overall well-being of your hair, you can contribute to the longevity and beauty of your locks. Striking a balance between style and hair health ensures that you not only look good but also feel good about the choices you make for your hair.

REGULAR TRIMS

Regular trims are a fundamental aspect of maintaining healthy, vibrant hair. In this extensive exploration, we will delve into the reasons why regular trims are crucial, the science behind them, the impact on different hair types, and practical tips for incorporating this proactive approach into your regular hair care routine.

The Significance of Regular Trims

Regular trims involve removing a small portion of the hair's length, typically every 6 to 12 weeks, depending on individual hair growth rates and preferences. While it might seem counterintuitive to cut hair to promote its growth, the benefits of regular trims are multifaceted and play a crucial role in overall hair health.

The Science Behind Regular Trims

Preventing Split Ends: Hair is susceptible to split ends, where the hair shaft splits into two or more parts. Regular trims help prevent split ends from traveling up the hair shaft, minimizing the need for more significant cuts later on.

Removing Damage: Hair can become damaged due to factors such as heat styling, chemical treatments, and environmental stressors. Regular trims remove damaged portions, promoting healthier and stronger hair.

Encouraging Growth: While trims don't directly increase the rate of hair growth, they create a healthier environment for hair to grow. By removing split ends and damage, the hair is less prone to breakage, allowing it to reach longer lengths over time.

Maintaining Shape and Style: For individuals with styled cuts or layers, regular trims help maintain the intended shape and style. This is essential for those who want to keep their hair looking polished and well-maintained.

The Impact of Regular Trims on Different Hair Types

Curly and Coily Hair: Curly and coily hair types are more prone to tangling and breakage. Regular trims help prevent split ends and maintain the overall health of these textured hair types.

Straight and Wavy Hair: Even straight and wavy hair benefits from regular trims to maintain a sleek appearance. Trims prevent the hair from looking dull and lifeless by removing damaged ends.

Fine and Thin Hair: Fine and thin hair types are more susceptible to breakage, and regular trims help minimize this risk. Keeping the ends healthy contributes to the overall volume and appearance of fine hair.

Chemically Treated Hair: Hair that has undergone chemical treatments, such as coloring or relaxing, is more prone to damage. Regular trims are essential for preserving the integrity of chemically treated hair and preventing further breakage.

Signs That You Need a Trim

Split Ends: If you notice split ends, it's an indication that your hair needs a trim. Ignoring split ends can lead to further damage and affect the overall health of your hair.

Dry and Brittle Ends: Dry and brittle ends are a sign of damage. Trimming these ends helps remove the damaged portions, allowing the hair to regain moisture and strength.

Tangling and Knots: Hair that frequently tangles and forms knots at the ends is likely in need of a trim. Removing damaged portions minimizes tangling and makes detangling more manageable.

Lack of Style Retention: If you have a styled cut or layers and notice that your hair isn't holding its shape, it might be time for a trim. Regular trims help maintain the intended style and structure.

Stalled Growth: If you feel like your hair growth has plateaued, it might be due to excessive breakage. Regular trims can address breakage issues, allowing your hair to grow more freely.

How to Trim Your Hair at Home

While professional trims are recommended for precision and expertise, occasional at-home trims can be done for maintenance between salon visits. Here's a basic guide for at-home trims:

Start with Clean, Dry Hair: Trimming dry, clean hair allows for more accurate length assessment. Comb your hair thoroughly to remove tangles.

Invest in Quality Hair Shears: Use sharp, quality hair shears designed for cutting hair. Avoid using regular household scissors, as they can cause additional damage.

Section Your Hair: Divide your hair into manageable sections. Clip away the sections you're not currently trimming to maintain focus and control.

Trim Small Sections: Take small sections of hair, about half an inch to an inch wide, and trim the tips. Focus on cutting the damaged or split ends.

Check for Evenness: Periodically check for evenness by comparing sections of your hair. This helps ensure a uniform trim.

Trim in a Straight Line: For a basic at-home trim, trim your hair in a straight line. If you have a specific style or layers, it's advisable to seek professional assistance.

Be Conservative: It's better to trim a little less than you think you need, especially if you're not experienced with cutting your own hair. You can always trim more if necessary.

Professional Haircuts and Trims

While at-home trims can be useful for maintenance, professional haircuts and trims are essential for achieving specific styles, addressing complex hair concerns, and ensuring precision. Here are some key considerations for professional trims:

Frequency: Visit a salon for a professional trim every 6 to 12 weeks, depending on your hair's needs and your desired style.

Consultation: Before the trim, communicate with your stylist about your hair goals, any specific concerns, and the desired outcome. A consultation helps ensure you and your stylist are on the same page.

STAY HYDRATED

Staying hydrated is a fundamental aspect of overall well-being, and its impact extends far beyond quenching thirst. In this comprehensive exploration, we will delve into the reasons why staying hydrated is crucial, the science behind hydration, the various factors influencing individual hydration needs, and practical tips for maintaining optimal hydration levels for enhanced health.

The Importance of Hydration

Biological Necessity:

The Science: Water is a vital component for numerous physiological processes within the body. It plays a crucial role in digestion, nutrient absorption, circulation, regulation of body temperature, and the elimination of waste products.
The Impact: Dehydration can disrupt these essential functions, leading to various health issues, including digestive problems, impaired kidney function, and difficulty maintaining a stable body temperature.

Cellular Function:

The Science: Cells require water to carry out their functions efficiently. Adequate hydration ensures optimal cell function, which is essential for overall

health, energy production, and the maintenance of organ systems.
The Impact: Dehydration at the cellular level can result in decreased energy levels, impaired cognitive function, and a compromised immune system.

Joint and Tissue Health:

The Science: Proper hydration is crucial for maintaining the lubrication of joints and supporting overall tissue health. Water is a key component in synovial fluid, which cushions and lubricates joints.
The Impact: Inadequate hydration may contribute to joint stiffness, reduced flexibility, and an increased risk of injuries related to joints and connective tissues.

Cognitive Function:

The Science: The brain is highly sensitive to changes in hydration status. Even mild dehydration can impair cognitive function, attention, and mood.
The Impact: Staying hydrated is essential for maintaining mental alertness, concentration, and overall cognitive performance.

Temperature Regulation:

The Science: Sweating is a crucial mechanism for regulating body temperature. When the body is dehydrated, the ability to sweat efficiently is compromised, leading to an increased risk of overheating.

The Impact: Inadequate hydration can result in heat-related illnesses, such as heat exhaustion or heatstroke, especially during physical activity or in hot environments.

Digestive Health:

The Science: Water is essential for the digestion and absorption of nutrients. It helps in breaking down food, transporting nutrients through the bloodstream, and aiding in the elimination of waste.

The Impact: Insufficient water intake can lead to constipation, indigestion, and an increased risk of gastrointestinal issues.

Factors Influencing Individual Hydration Needs

Body Weight:
Influence: Heavier individuals generally require more water than lighter individuals. Body weight is a key factor in determining the appropriate daily water intake.

Physical Activity:
Influence: Exercise increases fluid loss through sweating. Hydration needs are higher for those who engage in regular physical activity, especially intense or prolonged workouts.

Climate:

Influence: Hot and humid climates can lead to increased sweating and higher fluid loss. Individuals living in such climates need to adjust their hydration accordingly.

Age:
Influence: The hydration needs of infants, children, adults, and older adults can vary. Children and older adults may be more susceptible to dehydration and need to be mindful of their water intake.

Health Conditions:
Influence: Certain health conditions, such as kidney disease or diabetes, can affect fluid balance in the body. Individuals with specific medical conditions may have modified hydration requirements.

Pregnancy and Breastfeeding:
Influence: Pregnant and breastfeeding women have increased hydration needs to support fetal development and milk production.

Signs of Dehydration

Recognizing the signs of dehydration is crucial for addressing inadequate fluid intake promptly. Common signs include:

Dark Urine: Dark yellow or amber-colored urine can indicate dehydration. Adequately hydrated individuals typically have pale yellow urine.

Thirst: Thirst is a clear signal from the body that it needs more water. Responding to thirst cues is essential for maintaining hydration.

Dry Mouth and Skin: Dryness of the mouth and skin can be indicators of dehydration. Well-hydrated individuals generally have moist mucous membranes and supple skin.

Fatigue: Dehydration can lead to a decrease in energy levels and increased feelings of fatigue.

Headache: Headaches can be a symptom of dehydration. Proper hydration is essential for maintaining blood flow to the brain.

Dizziness or Lightheadedness: Inadequate fluid intake can result in dizziness or lightheadedness, especially when standing up.

Practical Tips for Staying Hydrated

Drink Water Throughout the Day:
Recommendation: Aim to sip water consistently throughout the day rather than consuming large amounts at once.

Listen to Your Body:
Recommendation: Pay attention to thirst cues. If you feel thirsty, drink water.

Carry a Reusable Water Bottle:
Recommendation: Having a water bottle on hand encourages regular sipping. Opt for a reusable bottle to reduce environmental impact.

Flavor Water Naturally:
Recommendation: Infuse water with natural flavors by adding slices of fruits, cucumbers, or herbs. This can make water more appealing without added sugars.

Set Hydration Goals:
Recommendation: Establish daily hydration goals based on individual needs, considering factors like body weight, activity level, and climate.

Include Hydrating Foods:
Recommendation: Consume water-rich foods such as fruits (watermelon, oranges) and vegetables (cucumbers, celery) to supplement fluid intake.

Monitor Urine Color:
Recommendation: Check the color of urine. Light yellow or pale straw color is a sign of adequate hydration.

Hydrate Before, During, and After Exercise:
Recommendation: Drink water before, during, and after physical activity to replenish fluids lost through sweating.

Limit Caffeine and Alcohol Intake:

Recommendation: Caffeine and alcohol can contribute to dehydration. Consume them in moderation and balance with water intake.

 Establish a Routine:
Recommendation: Incorporate regular water breaks into your daily routine, such as drinking a glass before meals.

Use Hydration Apps:
Recommendation: Utilize smartphone apps designed to track water intake and send reminders to stay hydrated.

REDUCE STRESS

Reducing stress is a crucial component of maintaining overall well-being and mental health. In this comprehensive exploration, we will delve into the reasons why stress reduction is essential, the physiological and psychological impact of stress, various stress management techniques, and practical tips for integrating stress reduction into daily life for a more balanced and healthy existence.

Understanding Stress

The Nature of Stress:

Definition: Stress is the body's natural response to challenges or threats, often referred to as the "fight or flight" response. It is a physiological and psychological reaction to situations perceived as demanding or harmful.
Impact: While stress is a normal part of life, chronic or excessive stress can have detrimental effects on physical and mental health.

Physiological Response:

Fight or Flight: When faced with a stressor, the body releases hormones such as cortisol and adrenaline. Heart rate increases, muscles tense, and other bodily functions prepare for immediate action.

Impact on the Body: While this response is crucial for survival in acute situations, prolonged activation of the stress response can contribute to various health issues.

Chronic Stress:

Definition: Chronic stress occurs when the stress response is continually activated over an extended period. It can result from ongoing challenges such as work pressures, financial concerns, or relationship issues.
Health Implications: Chronic stress has been linked to a range of health problems, including cardiovascular issues, compromised immune function, and mental health disorders.

Physiological and Psychological Impact

Cardiovascular Health:
Impact: Prolonged stress can contribute to high blood pressure, increased heart rate, and a higher risk of heart disease.

Immune System Function:
Impact: Chronic stress may suppress the immune system, making individuals more susceptible to infections and illnesses.

Mental Health:

Impact: Stress is a significant factor in the development and exacerbation of mental health conditions such as anxiety and depression.

Digestive Health:
Impact: Stress can affect the digestive system, leading to issues such as indigestion, irritable bowel syndrome (IBS), and other gastrointestinal problems.

Sleep Disruptions:
Impact: Stress can interfere with sleep patterns, contributing to insomnia or poor-quality sleep.

Cognitive Function:
Impact: Chronic stress may impair cognitive function, affecting memory, concentration, and decision-making.

Emotional Well-being:
Impact: Stress can contribute to mood swings, irritability, and feelings of overwhelm.

Stress Management Techniques

Mindfulness Meditation:
Technique: Mindfulness involves being fully present in the moment without judgment. Meditation practices, such as focused breathing or body scan meditations, can promote relaxation and reduce stress.

Deep Breathing Exercises:

Technique: Diaphragmatic or deep breathing involves slow, deep breaths to activate the body's relaxation response. This can be done through techniques like abdominal breathing or box breathing.

Progressive Muscle Relaxation (PMR):
Technique: PMR involves systematically tensing and then relaxing different muscle groups. This technique helps release physical tension associated with stress.

Yoga and Tai Chi:
Technique: Both yoga and tai chi combine physical movement, breath control, and mindfulness. Regular practice can enhance flexibility, balance, and stress resilience.

Exercise:
Technique: Regular physical activity, whether through aerobic exercise, strength training, or recreational activities, has been shown to reduce stress and improve mood.

Journaling:
Technique: Keeping a journal allows individuals to express their thoughts and feelings, providing a healthy outlet for processing stressors.

Cognitive-Behavioral Therapy (CBT):
Technique: CBT is a therapeutic approach that helps individuals identify and modify negative thought patterns and behaviors contributing to stress.

8. Social Support:
Technique: Maintaining strong social connections and seeking support from friends, family, or support groups can be instrumental in managing stress.

Time Management:
Technique: Effective time management can reduce feelings of overwhelm. Prioritizing tasks, setting realistic goals, and breaking them down into manageable steps can be helpful.

Art and Creativity:
Technique: Engaging in creative activities such as art, music, or writing can provide a therapeutic outlet for stress expression.

Aromatherapy:
Technique: Certain scents, such as lavender or chamomile, are believed to have calming effects. Aromatherapy using essential oils or scented candles can be incorporated into relaxation routines.